Keto Chaffle Cookbook for Your Lunch & Dinner

A Collection of Delicious Chaffle Recipes for Your Daily Meals

Kade Harrison

Table of Contents

5

Bacon Chaffle Omelettes

Servings: 2

Cooking Time:

10 Minutes

Ingredients:

- 2 slices bacon, raw
- 1 egg
- 1 tsp maple extract, optional
- 1 tsp all spices

Directions:

1. Put the bacon slices in a blender and turn it on.
2. Once ground up, add in the egg and all spices. Go on blending until liquefied.
3. Heat your waffle maker on the highest setting and spray with non-stick cooking spray.
4. Pour half the omelette into the waffle maker and cook for 5 minutes max.
5. Remove the crispy omelette and repeat the same steps with rest batter.

6. Enjoy warm.

Nutrition:

Calories per Servings: 59 Kcal ; Fats: 4.4 g ; Carbs: 1 g ; Protein: 5 g

Aioli Chicken Chaffle Sandwich

Servings: 1

Cooking Time:

6 Minutes

Ingredients:

- ¼ cup shredded rotisserie chicken
- 2 Tbsp Kewpie mayo
- ½ tsp lemon juice
- 1 grated garlic clove
- ¼ green onion, chopped
- 1 egg
- ½ cup shredded mozzarella cheese

Directions:

1. Mix lemon juice and mayo in a small bowl.
2. Turn on waffle maker to heat and oil it with cooking spray.
3. Beat egg in a small bowl.

4. Place ⅛ cup of cheese on waffle maker, then spread half of the egg mixture over it and top with ⅛ cup of cheese.
5. Close and cook for 3-minutes.
6. Repeat for remaining batter.
7. Place chicken on chaffles and top with sauce. Sprinkle with chopped green onion.

Nutrition:

Carbs: 3 g ;Fat: 42 g ;Protein: 34 g ;Calories: 545

Sage & Coconut Milk Chaffles

Servings: 6

Cooking Time:

24 Minutes

Ingredients:

- ¾ cup coconut flour, sifted
- 1½ teaspoons organic baking powder
- ½ teaspoon dried ground sage
- 1/8 teaspoon garlic powder
- 1/8 teaspoon salt
- 1 organic egg
- 1 cup unsweetened coconut milk
- ¼ cup water
- 1½ tablespoons coconut oil, melted
- ½ cup cheddar cheese, shredded

Directions:

1. Preheat a waffle iron and then grease it.
2. In a bowl, add the flour, baking powder, sage, garlic powder and salt and mix well.

3. Add the egg, coconut milk, water and coconut oil and mix until a stiff mixture forms.
4. Add the cheese and gently stir to combine.
5. Divide the mixture into 6 portions.
6. Place 1 portion of the mixture into preheated waffle iron and cook for about 4 minutes or until golden brown.
7. Repeat with the remaining mixture.
8. Serve warm.

Nutrition:

Calories: 147 Net Carb: 2.2g Fat: 13g Saturated Fat: 10.7g Carbohydrates: 2 Dietary Fiber: 0.7g Sugar: 1.3g Protein: 4g

Chaffle Burger

Servings: 1

Cooking Time:

10 Minutes

Ingredients:

- For the burger:
- ⅓-pound ground beef
- ½ tsp garlic salt
- 2 slices American cheese
- For the chaffles:
- 1 large egg
- ½ cup shredded mozzarella
- ¼ tsp garlic salt
- For the sauce:
- 2 tsp mayonnaise
- 1 tsp ketchup
- 1 tsp dill pickle relish
- splash vinegar, to taste
- For the toppings:
- 2 Tbsp shredded lettuce

- 3-4 dill pickles
- 2 tsp onion, minced

Directions:

1. Heat a griddle over medium-high heat.
2. Divide ground beef into balls and place on the griddle, 6 inches apart. Cook for 1 minute.
3. Use a small plate to flatten beef. Sprinkle with garlic salt.
4. Cook for 2-3, until halfway cooked through. Flip and sprinkle with garlic salt.
5. Cook for 2-3 minutes, or until cooked completely.
6. Place cheese slice over each patty and stack patties. Set aside on a plate. Cover with foil.
7. Turn on waffle maker to heat and oil it with cooking spray.
8. Whisk egg, cheese, and garlic salt until well combined.
9. Add half of the egg mixture to waffle maker and cook for 2-3 minutes.
10. Set aside and repeat with remaining batter.

11. Whisk all sauce ingredients in a bowl.

12. Top one chaffle with the stacked burger patties, shredded lettuce, pickles, and onions.

13. Spread sauce over the other chaffle and place sauce side down over the sandwich.

14. Eat immediately.

Nutrition:

Carbs: 8 g ;Fat: 56 g ;Protein: 65 g ;Calories: 831

Hot Ham Chaffles

Servings: 2

Cooking Time:

4 Minutes

Ingredients:

- ½ cup mozzarella cheese, shredded
- 1 egg
- ¼ cup ham, chopped
- ¼ tsp salt
- 2 tbsp mayonnaise
- 1 tsp Dijon mustard

Directions:

1. Preheat your waffle iron.
2. In the meantime, add the egg in a small mixing bowl and whisk.
3. Add in the ham, cheese, and salt. Mix to combine.
4. Scoop half the mixture using a spoon and pour into the hot waffle iron.

5. Close and cook for 4 minutes.

6. Remove the waffle and place on a large plate. Repeat the process with the remaining batter.

7. In a separate small bowl, add the mayo and mustard. Mix together until smooth.

8. Slice the waffles in quarters and use the mayo mixture as the dip.

Nutrition:

Calories per Servings: 110 Kcal ; Fats: 12 g ; Carbs: 6 g ; Protein: 12 g

Vegan Chaffle

Servings: 1

Cooking Time:

25 Minutes

Ingredients:

- 1 Tbsp flaxseed meal
- 2 ½ Tbsp water
- ¼ cup low carb vegan cheese
- 2 Tbsp coconut flour
- 1 Tbsp low carb vegan cream cheese, softened
- Pinch of salt

Directions:

1. Turn on waffle maker to heat and oil it with cooking spray.
2. Mix flaxseed and water in a bowl. Leave for 5 minutes, until thickened and gooey.
3. Whisk remaining ingredients for chaffle.

4. Pour one half of the batter into the center of the waffle maker. Close and cook for 3-5 minutes.
5. Remove chaffle and serve.

Nutrition:

Carbs: 33 g ;Fat: 25 g ;Protein: 25 g ;Calories: 450

Broccoli And Cheese Chaffles

Servings: 1

Cooking Time:

5 Minutes

Ingredients:

- ⅓ cup raw broccoli, finely chopped
- ¼ cup shredded cheddar cheese
- 1 egg
- ½ tsp garlic powder
- ½ tsp dried minced onion
- Salt and pepper, to taste

Directions:

1. Turn on waffle maker to heat and oil it with cooking spray.
2. Beat egg in a small bowl.
3. Fold in cheese, broccoli, onion, garlic powder, salt, and pepper.
4. Pour egg mixture into waffle maker. Cook for minutes, or until done.

5. Remove from waffle maker with a fork.

6. Serve with sour cream or butter.

Nutrition:

Carbs: 4 g ;Fat: 9 g ;Protein: g ;Calories: 125

Lemony Fresh Herbs Chaffles

Servings: 6

Cooking Time:

24 Minutes

Ingredients:

- ½ cup ground flaxseed
- 2 organic eggs
- ½ cup goat cheddar cheese, grated
- 2-4 tablespoons plain Greek yogurt
- 1 tablespoon avocado oil
- ½ teaspoon baking soda
- 1 teaspoon fresh lemon juice
- 2 tablespoons fresh chives, minced
- 1 tablespoon fresh basil, minced
- ½ tablespoon fresh mint, minced
- ¼ tablespoon fresh thyme, minced
- ¼ tablespoon fresh oregano, minced
- Salt and freshly ground black pepper, to taste

Directions:

1. Preheat a waffle iron and then grease it.
2. In a medium bowl, place all ingredients and with a fork, mix until well combined.
3. Divide the mixture into 6 portions.
4. Place 1 portion of the mixture into preheated waffle iron and cook for about minutes or until golden brown.
5. Repeat with the remaining mixture.
6. Serve warm.

Nutrition:

Calories: 11 Carb: 0.9g Fat: 7.9g Saturated Fat: 3g
Carbohydrates: 3.7g Dietary Fiber: 2.8g Sugar: 0.7g
Protein: 6.4g

Italian Seasoning Chaffles

Servings: 2

Cooking Time:

8 Minutes

Ingredients:

- ½ cup Mozzarella cheese, shredded
- 1 tablespoon Parmesan cheese, shredded
- 1 organic egg
- ¾ teaspoon coconut flour
- ¼ teaspoon organic baking powder
- 1/8 teaspoon Italian seasoning
- Pinch of salt

Directions:

1. Preheat a mini waffle iron and then grease it.
2. In a medium bowl, place all ingredients and with a fork, mix until well combined.
3. Place half of the mixture into preheated waffle iron and cook for about 4 minutes or until golden brown.

4. Repeat with the remaining mixture.

5. Serve warm.

Nutrition:

Calories: 8 Carb: 1.9g Fat: 5g Saturated Fat: 2.6g
Carbohydrates: 3.8g Dietary Fiber: 1.9g Sugar: 0.6g
Protein: 6.5g

Basil Chaffles

Servings: 3

Cooking Time: 1

6 Minutes

Ingredients:

- 2 organic eggs, beaten
- ½ cup Mozzarella cheese, shredded
- 1 tablespoon Parmesan cheese, grated
- 1 teaspoon dried basil, crushed
- Pinch of salt

Directions:

1. Preheat a mini waffle iron and then grease it.
2. In a medium bowl, place all ingredients and mix until well combined.
3. Place 1/of the mixture into preheated waffle iron and cook for about 3-4 minutes or until golden brown.
4. Repeat with the remaining mixture.
5. Serve warm.

Nutrition:

Calories: Net Carb: 0.4g Fat: 4.2g Saturated Fat: 1.6g Carbohydrates: 0.4g Dietary Fiber: 0g Sugar: 0.2g Protein: 5.7g

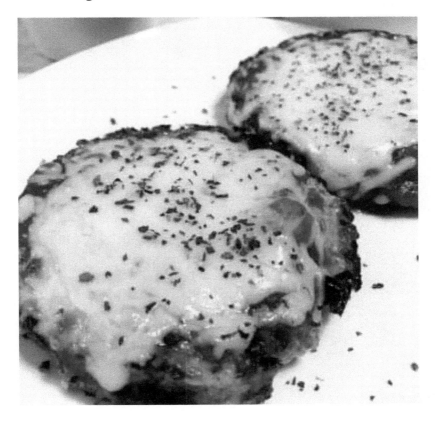

Bacon Chaffles

Servings: 2

Cooking Time:

5 Minutes

Ingredients:

- 2 eggs
- ½ cup cheddar cheese
- ½ cup mozzarella cheese
- ¼ tsp baking powder
- ½ Tbsp almond flour
- 1 Tbsp butter, for waffle maker
- For the filling:
- ¼ cup bacon, chopped
- 2 Tbsp green onions, chopped

Directions:

1. Turn on waffle maker to heat and oil it with cooking spray.

2. Add eggs, mozzarella, cheddar, almond flour, and baking powder to a blender and pulse 10 times, so cheese is still chunky.
3. Add bacon and green onions. Pulse 2-times to combine.
4. Add one half of the batter to the waffle maker and cook for 3 minutes, until golden brown.
5. Repeat with remaining batter.
6. Add your toppings and serve hot.

Nutrition:

Carbs: 3 g ;Fat: 38 g ;Protein: 23 g ;Calories: 446

Sausage Chaffles

Servings: 12

Cooking Time:

1 Hour

Ingredients:

- 1 pound gluten-free bulk Italian sausage, crumbled
- 1 organic egg, beaten
- 1 cup sharp Cheddar cheese, shredded
- ¼ cup Parmesan cheese, grated
- 1 cup almond flour
- 2 teaspoons organic baking powder

Directions:

1. Preheat a mini waffle iron and then grease it.
2. In a medium bowl, place all ingredients and with your hands, mix until well combined.
3. Place about 3 tablespoons of the mixture into preheated waffle iron and cook for about 3 minutes or until golden brown.

4. Carefully, flip the chaffle and cook for about 2 minutes or until golden brown.
5. Repeat with the remaining mixture.
6. Serve warm.

Nutrition:

Calories: 238 Net Carb: 1.2g Fat: 19.6g Saturated Fat: 6.1g Carbohydrates: 2.2g Dietary Fiber: 1g Sugar: 0.4g Protein: 10.8g

Scallion Cream Cheese Chaffle

Servings: 2

Cooking Time:

20 Minutes

Ingredients:

- 1 large egg
- ½ cup of shredded mozzarella
- 2 Tbsp cream cheese
- 1 Tbsp everything bagel seasoning
- 1-2 sliced scallions

Directions:

1. Turn on waffle maker to heat and oil it with cooking spray.
2. Beat egg in a small bowl.
3. Add in ½ cup mozzarella.
4. Pour half of the mixture into the waffle maker and cook for 3-minutes.
5. Remove chaffle and repeat with remaining mixture.

6. Let them cool, then cover each chaffle with cream cheese, sprinkle with seasoning and scallions.

Nutrition:

Carbs: 8 g ;Fat: 11 g ;Protein: 5 g ;Calories: 168

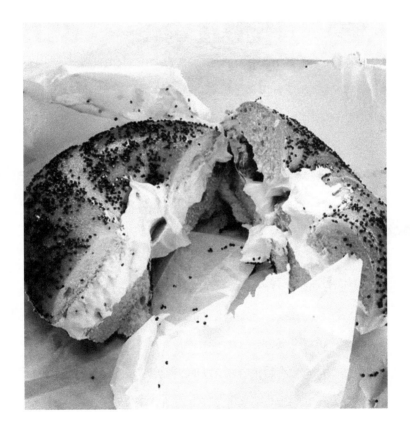

Broccoli Chaffles

Servings: 2

Cooking Time:

8 Minutes

Ingredients:

- 1/3 cup raw broccoli, chopped finely
- ¼ cup Cheddar cheese, shredded
- 1 organic egg
- ½ teaspoons garlic powder
- ½ teaspoons dried onion, minced
- Salt and freshly ground black pepper, to taste

Directions:

1. Preheat a mini waffle iron and then grease it.
2. In a medium bowl, place all ingredients and, mix until well combined.
3. Place ¼ of the mixture into preheated waffle iron and cook for about 4 minutes or until golden brown.
4. Repeat with the remaining mixture.

5. Serve warm.

Nutrition:

Calories: 9 Carb: 1.5g Fat: 6.9g Saturated Fat: 3.7g
Carbohydrates: 2g Dietary Fiber: 0.5g Sugar: 0.7g
Protein: 6.8g

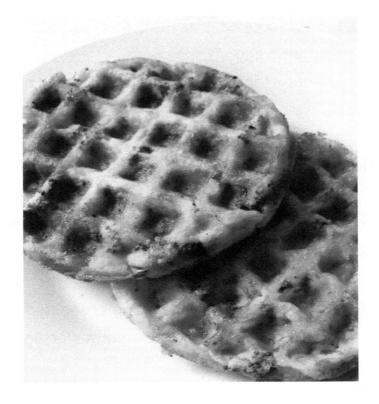

Chicken Taco Chaffles

Servings: 2

Cooking Time:

8 Minutes

Ingredients:

- 1/3 cup cooked grass-fed chicken, chopped
- 1 organic egg
- 1/3 cup Monterrey Jack cheese, shredded
- ¼ teaspoon taco seasoning

Directions:

1. Preheat a mini waffle iron and then grease it.
2. In a bowl, place all the ingredients and mix until well combined.
3. Place half of the mixture into preheated waffle iron and cook for about 4 minutes or until golden brown.
4. Repeat with the remaining mixture.
5. Serve warm.

Nutrition:

Calories: 141 Net Carb: 1.1g Fat: 8.9g Saturated Fat: 4.9g Carbohydrates: 1.1g Dietary Fiber: 0g Sugar: 0.2g Protein: 13.5g

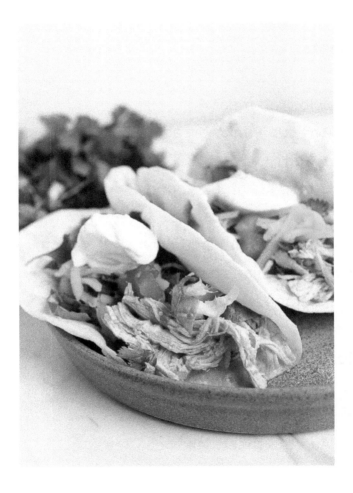

Crab Chaffles

Servings: 6

Cooking Time:

25 Minutes

Ingredients:

- 1 lb crab meat
- 1/3 cup Panko breadcrumbs
- 1 egg
- 2 tbsp fat greek yogurt
- 1 tsp Dijon mustard
- 2 tbsp parsley and chives, fresh
- 1 tsp Italian seasoning
- 1 lemon, juiced

Directions:

- Salt, pepper to taste
- Add the meat. Mix well.
- Form the mixture into round patties.
- Cook 1 patty for 3 minutes.

- Remove it and repeat the process with the remaining crab chaffle mixture.
- Once ready, remove and enjoy warm.

Nutrition:

Calories per Servings: 99 Kcal ; Fats: 8 g ; Carbs: 4 g ; Protein: 16 g

Bacon & 3-cheese Chaffles

Servings: 4

Cooking Time:

8 Minutes

Ingredients:

- 3 large organic eggs
- ½ cup Swiss cheese, grated
- 1/3 cup Parmesan cheese, grated
- 1/4 cup cream cheese, softened
- 4 tablespoons almond flour
- 1 tablespoon coconut flour
- ½ teaspoon onion powder
- ½ teaspoon garlic powder
- ½ teaspoon dried basil, crushed
- ½ teaspoon dried oregano, crushed
- ½ teaspoon organic baking powder
- Salt and freshly ground black pepper, to taste
- 4 cooked bacon slices, cut in half

Directions:

1. Preheat a waffle iron and then grease it.
2. In a bowl, place all the ingredients except for bacon and mix until well combined.
3. Place ¼ of the mixture into preheated waffle iron.
4. Arrange 2 halved bacon slices over mixture and cook for about 2 minutes or until golden brown.
5. Repeat with the remaining mixture and bacon slices.
6. Serve warm.

Nutrition:

Calories: 259 Net Carb: 3.2g Fat: 20.1g Saturated Fat: 8 Carbohydrates: 4.8g Dietary Fiber: 1.6g Sugar: 1g Protein: 13.9g

Spinach Chaffles

Servings: 4

Cooking Time:

20 Minutes

Ingredients:

- 1 large organic egg, beaten
- 1 cup ricotta cheese, crumbled
- ½ cup Mozzarella cheese, shredded
- ¼ cup Parmesan cheese, grated
- 4 ounces frozen spinach, thawed and squeezed
- 1 garlic clove, minced
- Salt and freshly ground black pepper, to taste

Directions:

1. Preheat a mini waffle iron and then grease it.
2. In a medium bowl, place all ingredients and mix until well combined.

3. Place ¼ of the mixture into preheated waffle iron and cook for about 4-5 minutes or until golden brown.
4. Repeat with the remaining mixture.
5. Serve warm.

Nutrition:

Calories: 139 Net Carb: 4.3g Fat: 8.1g Saturated Fat: 4g Carbohydrates: 4.7g Dietary Fiber: 0.4g Sugar: 0.4g Protein: 12.5g

Ground Beef Chaffles

Servings: 4

Cooking Time:

20 Minutes

Ingredients:

- ½ cup cooked grass-fed ground beef
- 3 cooked bacon slices, chopped
- 2 organic eggs
- ½ cup Cheddar cheese, shredded
- ½ cup Mozzarella cheese, shredded
- 2 teaspoons steak seasoning

Directions:

1. Preheat a mini waffle iron and then grease it.
2. In a medium bowl, place all ingredients and mix until well combined.
3. Place ¼ of the mixture into preheated waffle iron and cook for about 4-5 minutes or until golden brown.
4. Repeat with the remaining mixture.

5. Serve warm.

Nutrition:

Calories: 214 Net Carb: 0 g Fat: 12g Saturated Fat: 5.7g Carbohydrates: 0.5g Dietary Fiber: g Sugar: 0.2g Protein: 2.1g

Bacon & Egg Chaffles

Servings: 2

Cooking Time:

10 Minutes

Ingredients:

- 2 eggs
- 4 tsp collagen peptides, grass-fed
- 2 tbsp pork panko
- 3 slices crispy bacon

Directions:

1. Warm up your mini waffle maker.
2. Combine the eggs, pork panko, and collagen peptides. Mix well. Divide the batter in two small bowls.
3. Once done, evenly distribute ½ of the crispy chopped bacon on the waffle maker.
4. Pour one bowl of the batter over the bacon. Cook for 5 minutes and immediately repeat this step for the second chaffle.

5. Plate your cooked chaffles and sprinkle with extra Panko for an added crunch.
6. Enjoy!

Nutrition:

Calories per Servings: 266 Kcal ; Fats: 1g ; Carbs: 11.2 g ; Protein: 27 g

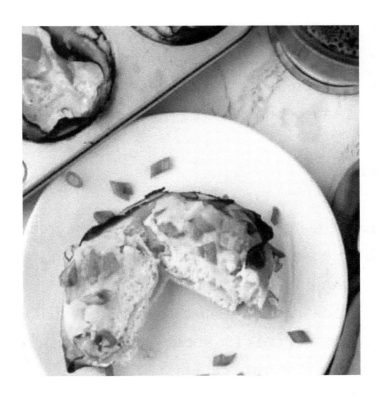

Chicken & Bacon Chaffles

Servings: 2

Cooking Time:

8 Minutes

Ingredients:

- 1 organic egg, beaten
- 1/3 cup grass-fed cooked chicken, chopped
- 1 cooked bacon slice, crumbled
- 1/3 cup Pepper Jack cheese, shredded
- 1 teaspoon powdered ranch dressing

Directions:

1. Preheat a mini waffle iron and then grease it.
2. In a medium bowl, place all ingredients and with a fork, mix until well combined.
3. Place half of the mixture into preheated waffle iron and cook for about 4 minutes or until golden brown.
4. Repeat with the remaining mixture.
5. Serve warm.

Nutrition:

Calories: 145 Net Carb: 0.9g Fat: 9.4g Saturated Fat: 4
Carbohydrates: 1g Dietary Fiber: 0.1g Sugar: 0.2g
Protein: 14.3g

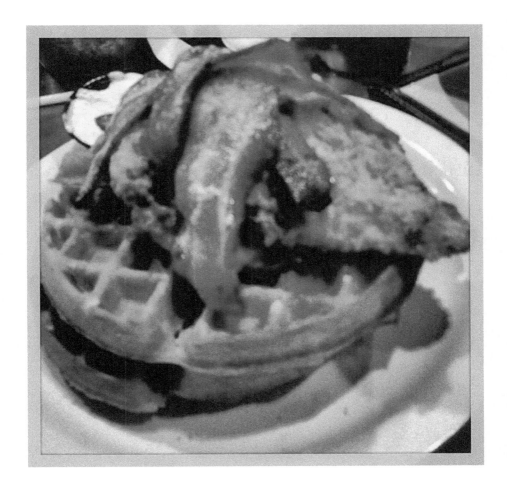

Belgium Chaffles

Servings: 1

Cooking Time:

6 Minutes

Ingredients:

- 2 eggs
- 1 cup Reduced-fat Cheddar cheese, shredded

Directions:

1. Turn on waffle maker to heat and oil it with cooking spray.
2. Whisk eggs in a bowl, add cheese. Stir until well-combined.
3. Pour mixture into waffle maker and cook for 6 minutes until done.
4. Let it cool a little to crisp before serving.

Nutrition:

Carbs: 2 g ;Fat: 33 g ;Protein: 44 g ;Calories: 460

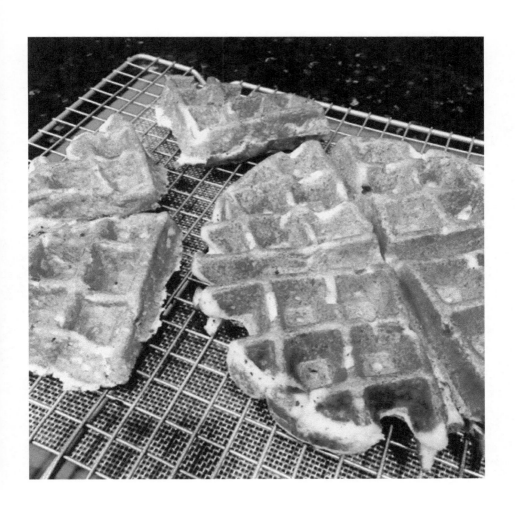

Salmon Chaffles

Servings: 2

Cooking Time:

10 Minutes

Ingredients:

- 1 large egg
- ½ cup shredded mozzarella
- 1 Tbsp cream cheese
- 2 slices salmon
- 1 Tbsp everything bagel seasoning

Directions:

1. Turn on waffle maker to heat and oil it with cooking spray.
2. Beat egg in a bowl, then add ½ cup mozzarella.
3. Pour half of the mixture into the waffle maker and cook for 4 minutes.
4. Remove and repeat with remaining mixture.

5. Let chaffles cool, then spread cream cheese, sprinkle with seasoning, and top with salmon.

Nutrition:

Carbs: 3 g ;Fat: 10 g ;Protein: 5 g ;Calories: 201

Chaffle Katsu Sandwich

Servings: 4

Cooking Time:

0 Minutes

Ingredients:

- For the chicken:
- ¼ lb boneless and skinless chicken thigh
- ⅛ tsp salt
- ⅛ tsp black pepper
- ½ cup almond flour
- 1 egg
- 3 oz unflavored pork rinds
- 2 cup vegetable oil for deep frying
- For the brine:
- 2 cup of water
- 1 Tbsp salt
- For the sauce:
- 2 Tbsp sugar-free ketchup
- 1½ Tbsp Worcestershire Sauce
- 1 Tbsp oyster sauce
- 1 tsp swerve/monkfruit

- For the chaffle:
- 2 egg
- 1 cup shredded mozzarella cheese

Directions:

1. Add brine ingredients in a large mixing bowl.
2. Add chicken and brine for 1 hour.
3. Pat chicken dry with a paper towel. Sprinkle with salt and pepper. Set aside.
4. Mix ketchup, oyster sauce, Worcestershire sauce, and swerve in a small mixing bowl.
5. Pulse pork rinds in a food processor, making fine crumbs.
6. Fill one bowl with flour, a second bowl with beaten eggs, and a third with crushed pork rinds.
7. Dip and coat each thigh in: flour, eggs, crushed pork rinds. Transfer on holding a plate.
8. Add oil to cover ½ inch of frying pan. Heat to 375°F.

9. Once oil is hot, reduce heat to medium and add chicken. Cooking time depends on the chicken thickness.

10. Transfer to a drying rack.

11. Turn on waffle maker to heat and oil it with cooking spray.

12. Beat egg in a small bowl.

13. Place ⅛ cup of cheese on waffle maker, then add¼ of the egg mixture and top with ⅛ cup of cheese.

14. Cook for 3-4 minutes.

15. Repeat for remaining batter.

16. Top chaffles with chicken katsu, 1 Tbsp sauce, and another piece of chaffle.

Nutrition:

Carbs: 12 g ;Fat: 1 g ;Protein: 2 g ;Calories: 57

Pork Rind Chaffles

Servings: 2

Cooking Time:

10 Minutes

Ingredients:

- 1 organic egg, beaten
- ½ cup ground pork rinds
- 1/3 cup Mozzarella cheese, shredded
- Pinch of salt

Directions:

1. Preheat a mini waffle iron and then grease it.
2. In a bowl, place all the ingredients and beat until well combined.
3. Place half of the mixture into preheated waffle iron and cook for about 5 minutes or until golden brown.
4. Repeat with the remaining mixture.
5. Serve warm.

Nutrition:

Calories: 91 Net Carb: 0.3g Fat: 5.9g Saturated Fat: 2.3g Carbohydrates: 0.3g Dietary Fiber: 0g Sugar: 0.2g Protein: 9.2g

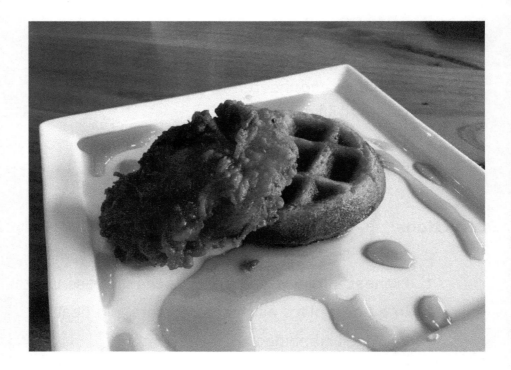

Chaffle Bruschetta

Servings: 1

Cooking Time:

5 Minutes

Ingredients:

- ½ cup shredded mozzarella cheese
- 1 whole egg beaten
- ¼ cup grated Parmesan cheese
- 1 tsp Italian Seasoning
- ¼ tsp garlic powder
- For the toppings:
- 3-4 cherry tomatoes, chopped
- 1 tsp fresh basil, chopped
- Splash of olive oil
- Pinch of salt

Directions:

1. Turn on waffle maker to heat and oil it with cooking spray.

2. Whisk all chaffle ingredients, except mozzarella, in a bowl.
3. Add in cheese and mix.
4. Add batter to waffle maker and cook for 5 minutes.
5. Mix tomatoes, basil, olive oil, and salt. Serve over the top of chaffles.

Nutrition:

Carbs: 2 g ;Fat: 24 g ;Protein: 34 g ;Calories: 352

Cheddar Protein Chaffles

Servings: 8

Cooking Time:

40 Minutes

Ingredients:

- ½ cup golden flax seeds meal
- ½ cup almond flour
- 2 tablespoons unsweetened whey protein powder
- 1 teaspoon organic baking powder
- Salt and freshly ground black pepper, to taste
- ¾ cup Cheddar cheese, shredded
- 1/3 cup unsweetened almond milk
- 2 tablespoons unsalted butter, melted
- 2 large organic eggs, beaten

Directions:

1. Preheat a mini waffle iron and then grease it.

2. In a large bowl, place flax seeds meal, flour, protein powder and baking powder and mix well.
3. Stir in the Cheddar cheese.
4. In another bowl, place the remaining ingredients and beat until well combined.
5. Add the egg mixture into the bowl with flax seeds meal mixture and mix until well combined.
6. Place desired amount of the mixture into preheated waffle iron and cook for about 4-5 minutes or until golden brown.
7. Repeat with the remaining mixture.
8. Serve warm.

Nutrition:

Calories: 187 Net Carb: 1.8g Fat: 14.5g Saturated Fat: 5g Carbohydrates: 4 Dietary Fiber: 3.1g Sugar: 0.4g Protein: 8g

Chicken & Ham Chaffles

Servings: 4

Cooking Time:

16 Minutes

Ingredients:

- ¼ cup grass-fed cooked chicken, chopped
- 1 ounce sugar-free ham, chopped
- 1 organic egg, beaten
- ¼ cup Swiss cheese, shredded
- ¼ cup Mozzarella cheese, shredded

Directions:

1. Preheat a mini waffle iron and then grease it.
2. In a medium bowl, place all ingredients and mix until well combined.
3. Place ¼ of the mixture into preheated waffle iron and cook for about 4 minutes or until golden brown.
4. Repeat with the remaining mixture.
5. Serve warm.

Nutrition:

Calories: 71 Net Carb: 0.7g Fat: 4.2g Saturated Fat: 2g
Carbohydrates: 0.8g Dietary Fiber: 0.1g Sugar: 0.2g
Protein: 7.4g

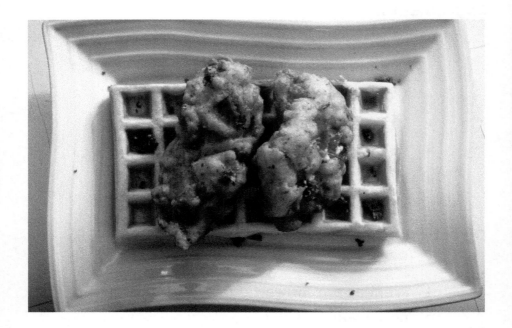

Herb Chaffles

Servings: 4

Cooking Time:

12 Minutes

Ingredients:

- 4 tablespoons almond flour
- 1 tablespoon coconut flour
- 1 teaspoon mixed dried herbs
- ½ teaspoon organic baking powder
- ¼ teaspoon garlic powder
- ¼ teaspoon onion powder
- Salt and ground black pepper, to taste
- ¼ cup cream cheese, softened
- 3 large organic eggs
- ½ cup cheddar cheese, grated
- 1/3 cup Parmesan cheese, grated

Directions:

1. Preheat a waffle iron and then grease it.

2. In a bowl, mix together the flours, dried herbs, baking powder, and seasoning, and mix well.
3. In a separate bowl, put cream cheese and eggs and beat until well combined.
4. Add the flour mixture, cheddar, and Parmesan cheese, and mix until well combined.
5. Place the desired amount of the mixture into preheated waffle iron and cook for about 2–3 minutes.
6. Repeat with the remaining mixture.
7. Serve warm.

Nutrition:

Calories 240 Net Carb: g Total Fat 19 g Saturated Fat 5 g Cholesterol 176 mg Sodium 280 mg Total Carbs 4 g Fiber 1.6 g Sugar 0.7 g Protein 12.3 g

Scallion Chaffles

Servings: 2

Cooking Time:

8 Minutes

Ingredients:

- 1 organic egg, beaten
- ½ cup Mozzarella cheese, shredded
- 1 tablespoon scallion, chopped
- ½ teaspoon Italian seasoning

Directions:

1. Preheat a mini waffle iron and then grease it.
2. In a medium bowl, place all ingredients and with a fork, mix until well combined.
3. Place half of the mixture into preheated waffle iron and cook for about 4 minutes or until golden brown.
4. Repeat with the remaining mixture.
5. Serve warm.

Nutrition:

Calories: 5 Carb: 0.7g Fat: 3.8g Saturated Fat: 1.5g
Carbohydrates: 0.8g Dietary Fiber: 0.g Sugar: 0.3g
Protein: 4.8g

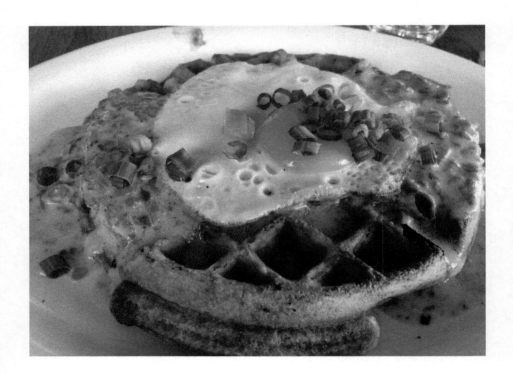

Eggs Benedict Chaffle

Servings: 2

Cooking Time:

10 Minutes

Ingredients:

- For the chaffle:
- 2 egg whites
- 2 Tbsp almond flour
- 1 Tbsp sour cream
- ½ cup mozzarella cheese
- For the hollandaise:
- ½ cup salted butter
- 4 egg yolks
- 2 Tbsp lemon juice
- For the poached eggs:
- 2 eggs
- 1 Tbsp white vinegar
- 3 oz deli ham

Directions:

1. Whip egg white until frothy, then mix in remaining ingredients.
2. Turn on waffle maker to heat and oil it with cooking spray.
3. Cook for 7 minutes until golden brown.
4. Remove chaffle and repeat with remaining batter.
5. Fill half the pot with water and bring to a boil.
6. Place heat-safe bowl on top of pot, ensuring bottom doesn't touch the boiling water.
7. Heat butter to boiling in a microwave.
8. Add yolks to double boiler bowl and bring to boil.
9. Add hot butter to the bowl and whisk briskly. Cook until the egg yolk mixture has thickened.
10.   Remove bowl from pot and add in lemon juice. Set aside.
11.   Add more water to pot if needed to make the poached eggs (water should completely cover the eggs). Bring to a simmer. Add white vinegar to water.

12.   Crack eggs into simmering water and cook
       for 1 minute 30 seconds. Remove using
       slotted spoon.

13.   Warm chaffles in toaster for 2-3 minutes.
       Top with ham, poached eggs, and hollandaise
       sauce.

Nutrition:

Carbs: 4 g ;Fat: 26 g ;Protein: 26 g ;Calories: 365

Chicken Bacon Chaffle

Servings: 2

Cooking Time:

5 Minutes

Ingredients:

- 1 egg
- ⅓ cup cooked chicken, diced
- 1 piece of bacon, cooked and crumbled
- ⅓ cup shredded cheddar jack cheese
- 1 tsp powdered ranch dressing

Directions:

1. Turn on waffle maker to heat and oil it with cooking spray.
2. Mix egg, dressing, and Monterey cheese in a small bowl.
3. Add bacon and chicken.
4. Add half of the batter to the waffle maker and cook for 3-minutes.

5. Remove and cook remaining batter to make a second chaffle.
6. Let chaffles sit for 2 minutes before serving.

Nutrition:

Carbs: 2 g ;Fat: 14 g ;Protein: 16 g ;Calories: 200

Bacon & Veggies Chaffles

Servings: 6

Cooking Time:

24 Minutes

Ingredients:

- 2 cooked bacon slices, crumbled
- ½ cup frozen chopped spinach, thawed and squeezed
- ½ cup cauliflower rice
- 2 organic eggs
- ½ cup Cheddar cheese, shredded
- ½ cup Mozzarella cheese, shredded
- ¼ cup Parmesan cheese, grated
- 1 tablespoon butter, melted
- 1 teaspoon garlic powder
- 1 teaspoon onion powder

Directions:

1. Preheat a mini waffle iron and then grease it.

2. In a bowl, place all the ingredients except blueberries and beat until well combined.
3. Fold in the blueberries.
4. Divide the mixture into 6 portions.
5. Place 1 portion of the mixture into preheated waffle iron and cook for about 3-4 minutes or until golden brown.
6. Repeat with the remaining mixture.
7. Serve warm.

Nutrition:

Calories: 10 Carb: 1.2gFat: 8.4g Saturated Fat: 4.6g Carbohydrates: 1.5g Dietary Fiber: 0.3g Sugar: 0.6g Protein: 7.1g

Garlic Cheese Chaffle Bread Sticks

Servings: 8

Cooking Time:

5 Minutes

Ingredients:

- 1 medium egg
- ½ cup mozzarella cheese, grated
- 2 Tbsp almond flour
- ½ tsp garlic powder
- ½ tsp oregano
- ½ tsp salt
- For the toppings:
- 2 Tbsp butter, unsalted softened
- ½ tsp garlic powder
- ¼ cup grated mozzarella cheese
- 2 tsp dried oregano for sprinkling

Directions:

1. Turn on waffle maker to heat and oil it with cooking spray.

2. Beat egg in a bowl.

3. Add mozzarella, garlic powder, flour, oregano, and salt, and mix.

4. Spoon half of the batter into the waffle maker.

5. Close and cook for minutes. Remove cooked chaffle.

6. Repeat with remaining batter.

7. Place chaffles on a tray and preheat the grill.

8. Mix butter with garlic powder and spread over the chaffles.

9. Sprinkle mozzarella over top and cook under the broiler for 2-3 minutes, until cheese has melted.

Nutrition:

Carbs: 1 g ;Fat: 7 g ;Protein: 4 g ;Calories: 74

Simple Savory Chaffles

Servings: 2

Cooking Time:

8 Minutes

Ingredients:

- 1 large organic egg, beaten
- ½ cup Cheddar cheese, shredded
- Pinch of salt and freshly ground black pepper

Directions:

1. Preheat a mini waffle iron and then grease it.
2. In a bowl, place all the ingredients and beat until well combined.
3. Place half of the mixture into preheated waffle iron and cook for about 4 minutes or until golden brown.
4. Repeat with the remaining mixture.
5. Serve warm.

Nutrition:

Calories: 150 Net Carb: 0 Fat: 11.9g Saturated Fat: 6.7g Carbohydrates: 0.6g Dietary Fiber: 0g Sugar: 0.3g Protein: 10.2g

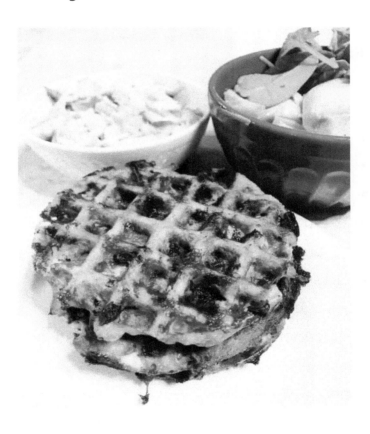

Parmesan Garlic Chaffle

Servings: 2

Cooking Time:

5 Minutes

Ingredients:

- 1 Tbsp fresh garlic minced
- 2 Tbsp butter
- 1-oz cream cheese, cubed
- 2 Tbsp almond flour
- 1 tsp baking soda
- 2 large eggs
- 1 tsp dried chives
- ½ cup parmesan cheese, shredded
- ¾ cup mozzarella cheese, shredded

Directions:

1. Heat cream cheese and butter in a saucepan over medium-low until melted.
2. Add garlic and cook, stirring, for minutes.

3. Turn on waffle maker to heat and oil it with cooking spray.
4. In a small mixing bowl, whisk together flour and baking soda, then set aside.
5. In a separate bowl, beat eggs for 1 minute 30 seconds on high, then add in cream cheese mixture and beat for 60 seconds more.
6. Add flour mixture, chives, and cheeses to the bowl and stir well.
7. Add ¼ cup batter to waffle maker.
8. Close and cook for 4 minutes, until golden brown.
9. Repeat for remaining batter.
10.   Add favorite toppings and serve.

Nutrition:

Carbs: 5 g ;Fat: 33 g ;Protein: 19 g ;Calories: 385

Chicken & Veggies Chaffles

Servings: 3

Cooking Time:

15 Minutes

Ingredients:

- 1/3 cup cooked grass-fed chicken, chopped
- 1/3 cup cooked spinach, chopped
- 1/3 cup marinated artichokes, chopped
- 1 organic egg, beaten
- 1/3 cup Mozzarella cheese, shredded
- 1 ounce cream cheese, softened
- ¼ teaspoon garlic powder

Directions:

1. Preheat a mini waffle iron and then grease it.
2. In a medium bowl, place all ingredients and mix until well combined.
3. Place 1/of the mixture into preheated waffle iron and cook for about 4-5 minutes or until golden brown.

4. Repeat with the remaining mixture.

5. Serve warm.

Nutrition:

Calories: 95 Net Carb: 1.3g Fat: 5.8g Saturated Fat: 1.3g Carbohydrates: 2.2g Dietary Fiber: 0.9g Sugar: 0.3g Protein: 8.

Turkey Chaffles

Servings: 4

Cooking Time:

16 Minutes

Ingredients:

- ½ cup cooked turkey meat, chopped
- 2 organic eggs, beaten
- ½ cup Parmesan cheese, grated
- ½ cup Mozzarella, shredded
- ¼ teaspoon poultry seasoning
- ¼ teaspoon onion powder

Directions:

1. Preheat a mini waffle iron and then grease it.
2. In a medium bowl, place all ingredients and mix until well combined.
3. Place ¼ of the mixture into preheated waffle iron and cook for about 4 minutes or until golden brown.

4. Repeat with the remaining mixture.

5. Serve warm.

Nutrition:

Calories: 108 Net Carb: 0.5g Fat: 1g Saturated Fat: 2.6g Carbohydrates: 0.5g Dietary Fiber: 0g Sugar: 0.2g Protein: 12.9g

Chicken & Zucchini Chaffles

Servings: 9

Cooking Time:

0 Minutes

Ingredients:

- 4 ounces cooked grass-fed chicken, chopped
- 2 cups zucchini, shredded and squeezed
- ¼ cup scallion, chopped
- 2 large organic eggs
- ½ cup Mozzarella cheese, shredded
- ½ cup Cheddar cheese, shredded
- ½ cup blanched almond flour
- 1 teaspoon organic baking powder
- ½ teaspoon garlic salt
- ½ teaspoon onion powder

Directions:

1. Preheat a waffle iron and then grease it.
2. In a medium bowl, place all ingredients and mix until well combined.

3. Divide the mixture into 9 portions.

4. Place 1 portion of the mixture into preheated waffle iron and cook for about 2-3 minutes or until golden brown.

5. Repeat with the remaining mixture.

6. Serve warm.

Nutrition:

Calories: 108 Net Carb: 2g Fat: 6.9g Saturated Fat: 2.2g Carbohydrates: 3.1g Dietary Fiber: 1.1g Sugar: 0 Protein: 8.8g

Pepperoni Chaffles

Servings: 1

Cooking Time:

5 Minutes

Ingredients:

- 1 organic egg, beaten
- ½ cup Mozzarella cheese, shredded
- 2 tablespoons turkey pepperoni slice, chopped
- 1 tablespoon sugar-free pizza sauce
- ¼ teaspoon Italian seasoning

Directions:

1. Preheat a waffle iron and then grease it.
2. In a bowl, place all the ingredients and mix well.
3. Place the mixture into preheated waffle iron and cook for about 5 minutes or until golden brown.
4. Serve warm.

Nutrition:

Calories: 119 Net Carb: 2.4gFat: 7g Saturated Fat: 3g
Carbohydrates: 2.7g Dietary Fiber: 0.3g Sugar: 0.9g
Protein: 10.3g

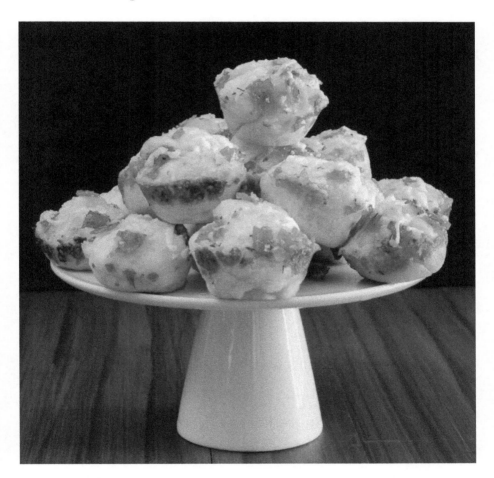

Hot Sauce Jalapeño Chaffles

Servings: 2

Cooking Time:

8 Minutes

Ingredients:

- ½ cup plus 2 teaspoons Cheddar cheese, shredded and divided
- 1 organic egg, beaten
- 6 jalapeño pepper slices
- ¼ teaspoon hot sauce
- Pinch of salt

Directions:

1. Preheat a mini waffle iron and then grease it.
2. In a bowl, place ½ cup of cheese and remaining ingredients and mix until well combined.
3. Place about 1 teaspoon of cheese in the bottom of the waffle maker for about seconds before adding the mixture.

4. Place half of the mixture into preheated waffle iron and cook for about 3-minutes or until golden brown.
5. Repeat with the remaining cheese and mixture.
6. Serve warm.

Nutrition:

Calories: 153 Net Carb: 0.6g Fat: 12.2gSaturated Fat: Carbohydrates: 0.7g Dietary Fiber: 0.1g Sugar: 0.4g Protein: 10.3g

Chicken Chaffles

Servings: 4

Cooking Time:

15 Minutes

Ingredients:

- 2 oz chicken breasts, cooked, shredded
- 1/2 cup mozzarella cheese, finely shredded
- 2 eggs
- 6 tbsp parmesan cheese, finely shredded
- 1 cup zucchini, grated
- ½ cup almond flour
- 1tsp baking powder
- ¼ tsp garlic powder
- ¼ tsp black pepper, ground
- ½ tsp Italian seasoning
- ¼ tsp salt

Directions:

1. Sprinkle the zucchini with a pinch of salt and set it aside for a few minutes. Squeeze out the excess water.

2. Warm up your mini waffle maker.
3. Mix chicken, almond flour, baking powder, cheeses, garlic powder, salt, pepper and seasonings in a bowl.
4. Use another small bow for beating eggs. Add them to squeezed zucchini, mix well.
5. Combine the chicken and egg mixture, and mix.
6. For a crispy crust, add a teaspoon of shredded cheese to the waffle maker and cook for 30 seconds.
7. Then, pour the mixture into the waffle maker and cook for 5 minutes or until crispy.
8. Carefully remove. Repeat with remaining batter the same steps.
9. Enjoy!

Nutrition:

Calories per Servings: 135 Kcal ; Fats: g ; Carbs: 3 g ; Protein: 11 g

Garlicky Chicken Chaffles

Servings: 2

Cooking Time:

12 Minutes

Ingredients:

- 1 organic egg, beaten
- 1/3 cup grass-fed cooked chicken, chopped
- 1/3 cup Mozzarella cheese, shredded
- ¼ teaspoon garlic, minced
- ¼ teaspoon dried basil, crushed

Directions:

1. Preheat a mini waffle iron and then grease it.
2. In a bowl, place all the ingredients and mix until well combined.
3. Place half of the mixture into preheated waffle iron and cook for about 4-6 minutes or until golden brown.
4. Repeat with the remaining mixture.
5. Serve warm.

Nutrition:

Calories: 81 Net Carb: 0.5g Fat: 3.7g Saturated Fat: 1.4g Carbohydrates: 0.5g Dietary Fiber: 0g Sugar: 0.2g Protein: 10.9g

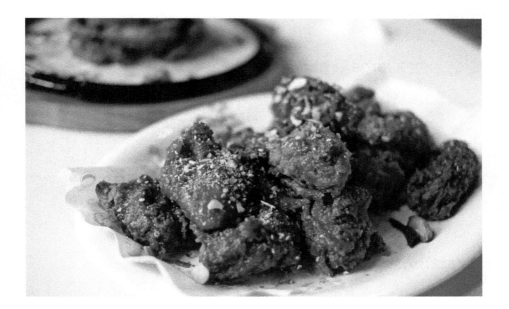

Garlic Herb Blend Seasoning Chaffles

Servings: 2

Cooking Time:

8 Minutes

Ingredients:

- 1 large organic egg, beaten
- ¼ cup Parmesan cheese, shredded
- ¼ cup Mozzarella cheese, shredded
- ½ tablespoon butter, melted
- 1 teaspoon garlic herb blend seasoning
- Salt, to taste

Directions:

1. Preheat a mini waffle iron and then grease it.
2. In a bowl, place all the ingredients and beat until well combined.
3. Place half of the mixture into preheated waffle iron and cook for about 4 minutes or until golden brown.
4. Repeat with the remaining mixture.

5. Serve warm.

Nutrition:

Calories: 115 Net Carb: 1.1g Fat: 8.8g Saturated Fat: 4.7g Carbohydrates: 1.2g Dietary Fiber: 0.1g Sugar: 0.2g Protein: 8g

Protein Cheddar Chaffles

Servings: 8

Cooking Time:

48 Minutes

Ingredients:

- ½ cup golden flax seeds meal
- ½ cup almond flour
- 2 tablespoons unflavored whey protein powder
- 1 teaspoon organic baking powder
- Salt and ground black pepper, to taste
- ¾ cup cheddar cheese, shredded
- 1/3 cup unsweetened almond milk
- 2 tablespoons unsalted butter, melted
- 2 large organic eggs, beaten

Directions:

1. Preheat a mini waffle iron and then grease it.
2. In a large bowl, add flax seeds meal, flour, protein powder, and baking powder, and mix well.

3. Stir in the cheddar cheese.
4. In another bowl, add the remaining ingredients and beat until well combined.
5. Add the egg mixture into the bowl with flax seeds meal mixture and mix until well combined.
6. Place desired amount of the mixture into preheated waffle iron.
7. Cook for about 4–6 minutes.
8. Repeat with the remaining mixture.
9. Serve warm.

Nutrition:

Calories 187 Net Carbs 1.8 g Total Fat 14.5 g Saturated Fat 5 g Cholesterol 65 mg Sodium 134 mg Total Carbs 4.9 g Fiber 3.1 g Sugar 0.4 g Protein 8 g

Garlic & Onion Powder Chaffles

Servings: 1

Cooking Time:

5 Minutes

Ingredients:

- 1 organic egg, beaten
- ¼ cup Cheddar cheese, shredded
- 2 tablespoons almond flour
- ½ teaspoon organic baking powder
- ¼ teaspoon garlic powder
- ¼ teaspoon onion powder
- Pinch of salt

Directions:

1. Preheat a waffle iron and then grease it.
2. In a bowl, place all the ingredients and beat until well combined.

3. Place the mixture into preheated waffle iron and cook for about 5 minutes or until golden brown.
4. Serve warm.

Nutrition:

Calories: 274 Net Carb: 3.3g Fat: 21.3g Saturated Fat: 7.8g Dietary Fiber: 1.7g Sugar: 1.4g Protein: 12.8g

Cheese-free Breakfast Chaffle

Servings: 1

Cooking Time:

12 Minutes

Ingredients:

- 1 egg
- ½ cup almond milk ricotta, finely shredded.
- 1 tbsp almond flour
- 2 tbsp butter

Directions:

1. Mix the egg, almond flour and ricotta in a small bowl.
2. Separate the chaffle batter into two and cook each for 4 minutes.
3. Melt the butter and pour on top of the chaffles.
4. Put them back in the pan and cook on each side for 2 minutes.

5. Remove from the pan and allow them sit for 2 minutes.
6. Enjoy while still crispy.

Nutrition:

Calories: 530 Kcal ; Fats: 50 g ; Carbs: 3 g ; Protein: 23 g

Savory Bagel Seasoning Chaffles

Servings:4

Cooking Time:

5 Minutes

Ingredients:

- 2 tbsps. everything bagel seasoning
- 2 eggs
- 1 cup mozzarella cheese
- 1/2 cup grated parmesan

Directions:

1. Preheat the square waffle maker and grease with cooking spray.
2. Mix together eggs, mozzarella cheese and grated cheese in a bowl.
3. Pour half of the batter in the waffle maker.
4. Sprinkle 1 tbsp. of the everything bagel seasoning over batter.
5. Close the lid.
6. Cook chaffles for about 3-4 minutesutes.

7. Repeat with the remaining batter.

8. Serve hot and enjoy!

Nutrition:

Protein: 34% 71 kcal Fat: 60% 125 kcal Carbohydrates: 6% 13 kcal

Dried Herbs Chaffles

Servings: 2

Cooking Time:

8 Minutes

Ingredients:

- 1 organic egg, beaten
- ½ cup Cheddar cheese, shredded
- 1 tablespoon almond flour
- Pinch of dried thyme, crushed
- Pinch of dried rosemary, crushed

Directions:

1. Preheat a mini waffle iron and then grease it.
2. In a bowl, place all the ingredients and beat until well combined.
3. Place half of the mixture into preheated waffle iron and cook for about 4 minutes or until golden brown.
4. Repeat with the remaining mixture.
5. Serve warm.

Nutrition:

Calories: 1 Net Carb: 0.9g Fat: 13.4g Saturated Fat: 6.8g Carbohydrates: 1.3g Dietary Fiber: 0.4g Sugar: 0.4g Protein: 9.8g

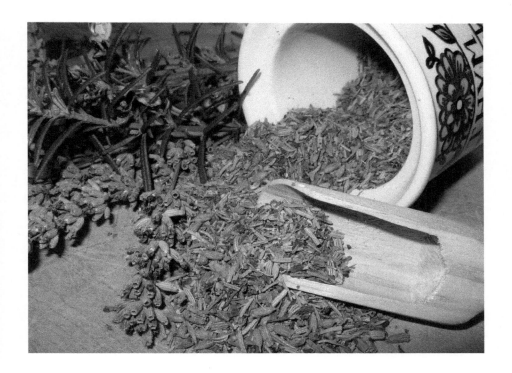

Sour Cream Protein Chaffles

Servings: 4

Cooking Time:

16 Minutes

Ingredients:

- 6 organic eggs
- ½ cup sour cream
- ½ cup unsweetened whey protein powder
- 1 teaspoon organic baking powder
- ½ teaspoon salt
- 1 cup Cheddar cheese, shredded

Directions:

1. Preheat a waffle iron and then grease it.
2. In a medium bowl, place all ingredients and mix until well combined.
3. Place ¼ of the mixture into preheated waffle iron and cook for about 4 minutes or until golden brown.
4. Repeat with the remaining mixture.

5. Serve warm.

Nutrition:

Calories: 324Net Carb: 3 Fat: 22.6g Saturated Fat: 11.9g Carbohydrates: 3.6g Dietary Fiber: 0g Sugar: 1.3g Protein: 27.3g

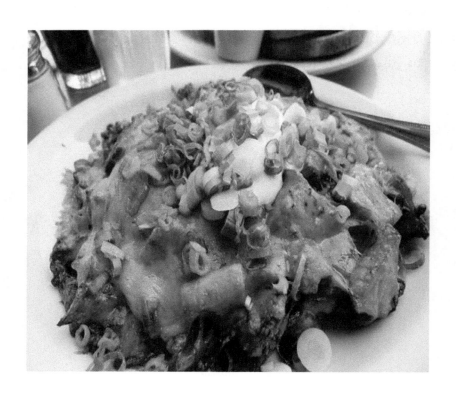